Asthma
Second Edition

Peter J Barnes, DM, DSc, FRCP
Professor of Thoracic Medicine
National Heart and Lung Institute
Imperial College School of Medicine
London, UK

Simon Godfrey, MD, PhD, FRCP
Professor of Pediatrics
Director, Institute of Pulmonology
Hadassah University Hospital
Jerusalem, Israel

MARTIN DUNITZ

© Martin Dunitz Ltd 1995, 1996, 2000

First published in the United Kingdom
in 1995 by
Martin Dunitz Ltd
The Livery House
7– 9 Pratt Street
London NW1 0AE

Revised edition 1996
Second edition 2000

A CIP record for this book is available
from the British Library.

ISBN 1-85317-667-2

Printed and bound in Spain by Cayfosa

Contents

What is asthma?

Definitions

Asthma is a syndrome characterized by airflow obstruction that varies markedly, both spontaneously and with treatment.

There is a special type of inflammation in the airways which makes them hyperresponsive to a wide range of triggers, so that they narrow excessively. Narrowing of the airways is usually reversible, but in some patients with chronic asthma there may be an element of irreversible airflow obstruction.

Epidemiological trends

- Asthma affects approximately 10–15% of children and 5–10% of adults
- Asthma prevalence is greater in industrialized countries but differences with developing countries are lessening
- The prevalence of asthma is increasing world-wide
- Until recently hospital admissions with asthma were steadily increasing
- Asthma mortality has not decreased significantly, despite improvements in management. However, in relation to the frequency of hospital admissions mortality has fallen

Cont'd.

- Prescribed therapy for asthma is increasing (especially inhaled β_2-agonists)
- The reasons for the world-wide increase in asthma morbidity and mortality are unknown

Pathology of asthma

The airways show a characteristic pathology which varies in intensity from mild to fatal asthma (Fig. 1). Characteristics are:

- Infiltration with inflammatory cells (especially eosinophils and T-lymphocytes)
- Patchy epithelial shedding
- Airway smooth muscle thickening
- Subepithelial fibrosis
- Mucus gland and goblet cell hyperplasia
- Widespread mucus plugging in fatal and severe asthma

Mechanisms of asthma

- Fibreoptic bronchial biopsies have shown that inflammation is present even in patients with mild asthma who are asymptomatic
- Inflammation underlies airway hyperresponsiveness: an increased airway narrowing in response to a wide range of stimuli (including mediators and physical stimuli) (Fig. 2)
- There is a characteristic pattern of inflammation, with activated mast cells, macrophages, eosinophils and T-helper lymphocytes ('chronic eosinophilic bronchitis') (Fig. 3)
- Inflammatory cells release multiple inflammatory mediators (including histamine, leukotrienes, prostaglandins and bradykinin)
- Multiple intracellular messengers called cytokines (e.g. interleukin-1, interleukin-5) are responsible for coordinating, amplifying and perpetuating the inflammatory response and attracting additional inflammatory cells

- Inflammatory mediators result in bronchoconstriction, mucus secretion, exudation of plasma and airway hyperresponsiveness
- Neural mechanisms may amplify the asthmatic inflammation (neurogenic inflammation)
- Structural changes may occur with subepithelial fibrosis (basement membrane thickening), airway smooth muscle hyperplasia and new vessel formation. These changes may underlie irreversible (fixed) airflow obstruction

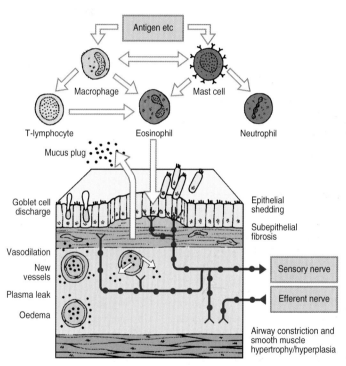

Figure 1
Asthma is a complex inflammatory disease involving many inflammatory cells which interact, releasing multiple inflammatory mediators that cause bronchoconstriction and complex inflammatory effects on the airways.

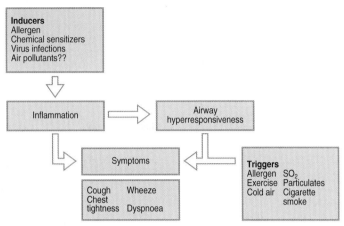

Figure 2
Relationship between airway inflammation, airway hyperresponsiveness and symptoms of asthma.

Types of asthma

Several clinical types of asthma are recognized, although the pathological appearances are similar.

Allergic (extrinsic) asthma: in atopic patients
Onset usually in childhood and may persist into adulthood, although remission in adolescence is common. Associated with allergic rhinitis and atopic dermatitis (eczema)

Non-allergic (intrinsic) asthma: non-atopic patients
Onset in adults (late-onset asthma). Often associated with perennial non-allergic rhinitis. Accounts for approximately 10% of adult asthma. There is a special (relatively rare) type of intrinsic asthma in which the patient is exquisitely sensitive to aspirin and other non-steroidal anti-inflammatory drugs (NSAIDS)

Occupational asthma
Due to exposure to chemical sensitizers (e.g. toluene diisocyanate) at work. Unrelated to atopic status. Some occupational asthmas occur in atopic subjects due to allergen exposure at work

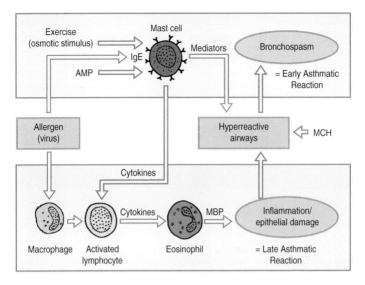

Figure 3
Diagrammatic representation of the mechanisms leading to early and late phase asthmatic reactions. The central abnormality is bronchial hyperreactivity which is the result of chronic asthmatic inflammatory changes and epithelial damage in the airways. When mast cells are stimulated allergically or by other means such as exercise or adenosine monophosphate (AMP) they liberate mediators which cause bronchospasm (the early type of reaction). Allergic stimulation and other mechanisms (such as viral infection) can also initiate lymphocyte activation and cytokine release which leads to inflammatory infiltration (the late type of reaction) and epithelial damage in which eosinophils are involved. Hyperreactive airways from any cause, including for example COPD, can respond to direct stimulation by methacholine (MCH).

Causes of asthma

The underlying causes of asthma are not known. Atopy (the propensity to form IgE) is inherited, but environmental mechanisms appear to be important in determining whether an atopic individual becomes asthmatic. Several factors may increase the risks of developing asthma:

- Maternal smoking (in pregnancy and infancy)
- Exposure to a high concentration of allergens (e.g. house dust mite)
- Some studies suggest a lack of early childhood infections may predispose to the development of asthma but viral infection during infancy (especially respiratory syncytial virus) may initiate the disease. Further data are required to clarify this point.
- Air pollution (ozone, SO_2, NO_2): no convincing evidence

Natural history of asthma

Because asthma is both common and frequently complicated by the effects of smoking on the lungs it is difficult to be certain about the natural history of the disease in adults. Patients with late onset asthma rarely lose the disease although its severity may fluctuate with a corresponding change in management requirements. The picture in children is clearer and the commonly held belief that children 'grow out of their asthma' is justified to some extent. Long-term studies which have followed children until they reach 30–40 years of age suggest about two thirds of asthmatic children become asymptomatic in childhood and remain so at least until mid-adult life; about one sixth become asymptomatic only to have the disease return in adult life; about one sixth never become asymptomatic.

There is some evidence that effective early introduction of anti-inflammatory treatment in children with asthma improves the prognosis in the sense that the earlier the treatment is started, the greater the improvement in lung function. Although there is a clinical impression that children are 'growing out' of their asthma sooner since the introduction of effective anti-inflammatory treatment at an earlier stage this has not yet been subjected to formal evaluation.

Clinical features

Symptoms

Asthma symptoms may vary in intensity and some symptoms may be more prominent in some patients.

- Wheeze: intermittent, worse on expiration, characteristically relieved by an inhaled β_2-agonist
- Cough: usually unproductive. May be presenting symptom (especially in children)
- Chest tightness
- Shortness of breath (not always associated with wheeze)
- Sputum production (usually scanty)
- Prodromal symptoms may precede an attack: itching under the chin, discomfort between shoulder blades, inexplicable fear

Triggers

Several factors may trigger asthma symptoms and should be elicited in the history.

- Allergens (house dust mite, pollen, animal dander, moulds, cockroach)
- Irritants (tobacco smoke, air pollutants, strong odours, fumes)
- Physical factors (exercise, cold air, hyperventilation, laughter, crying)
- Upper respiratory tract viral infections
- Emotions (stress)
- Occupational agents (chemical sensitizers, allergens)
- Drugs (β-blockers, non-steroidal anti-inflammatory drugs)
- Food additives (metabisulphite, tartrazine?)
- Change in weather
- Endocrine factors (menstrual cycle, pregnancy, thyroid disease)
- Time of day (during the night or usually early morning)

Physical signs

Physical examination in asthma may be normal. Characteristic signs may include:

- Expiratory rhonchi (widespread); intensity may not be related to severity
- Hyperinflation of chest, use of accessory muscles, chest deformity in children with chronic poorly controlled asthma (pigeon chest)
- Crackles/crepitations (espcially in young children)
- Associated signs: nasal polyps, flexural eczema

Investigations

Lung function tests

Lung function tests are essential to document the severity of asthma. Simple tests performed repeatedly are more useful than complex tests. Normal values of lung function are given in Figs 17–20.

Spirometry

The hallmark of asthma is its variability and it is therefore to be expected that the lung function of the patient will also vary. For most asthmatics, this variability is so marked over relatively short periods of time that the infrequent measurement of lung function is all but useless in evaluating the overall status of the patient. In many situations, it is adequate for lung function to be measured whenever the patient attends the asthma clinic provided he is seen relatively frequently and his clinical control is good. While there are a variety of sophisticated tests of lung function, the most informative is a forced expiratory spirogram taken before and after the inhalation of a bronchodilator.

Nowadays it is usual for electronic spirometers to provide the results as both volume–time and flow–volume plots (Fig. 4) which show exactly the same data in different formats. The following are the most useful indices obtained from the spirogram:

Forced vital capacity (FVC): the total volume that can be expelled during a maximal effort after maximal inspiration. This should be normal for the sex, age and height of the patient, except in moderate to severe asthma when it may be reduced because of gas trapping which prevents expiration to normal levels. It may also be reduced because of lack of cooperation by the patient as it is a very effort-dependent test.

Forced expired volume in 1 second (FEV_1): the volume that is expelled in the first second of the forced expiration . This is the most useful overall index of lung function in asthmatics and reflects the global severity of the airways obstruction. It is relatively independent of effort provided the patient makes a reasonable attempt to expel the air rapidly. It should be compared with the predicted value which is usually given in the print-out of results by the spirometer. A reduced FEV_1/FVC ratio (<75%) is often taken as an index of the severity of

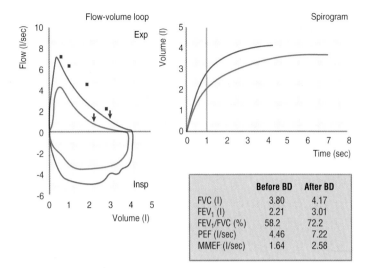

	Before BD	After BD
FVC (l)	3.80	4.17
FEV$_1$ (l)	2.21	3.01
FEV$_1$/FVC (%)	58.2	72.2
PEF (l/sec)	4.46	7.22
MMEF (l/sec)	1.64	2.58

Figure 4
Lung function in a patient with asthma. The blue lines are the baseline measurements, and the pink lines show improvement after inhalation of a bronchodilator (salbutamol 200 μg). Left panel shows flow-volume loops with inspiratory and expiratory records. Squares indicate the predicted normal value of the expiratory loop and arrows indicate the volume expired after 1 second. Right panel shows the expiratory spirogram for the same breath. The dashed line indicates the volumes at 1 second. The results of the test are shown below and indicate generalized airflow obstruction with improvement (36% increase in FEV$_1$) after bronchodilator.

airways obstruction. Since the FVC is so effort-dependent and is itself reduced in severe asthma, this ratio is potentially misleading.

Peak expiratory flow (PEF): the maximum expiratory flow achieved during forced expiration — usually within the first few milliseconds of the expiratory effort. This is the simplest test of lung function and can also be measured with simple devices in the home. It is very effort-dependent but quite reproducible in patients who cooperate fully with the test. The PEF reflects chiefly the severity of obstruction in the larger airways and its main disadvantage is that it can be totally normal when the patient has marked small airways obstruction.

Maximum mid-expiratory flow (MMEF): the maximum expiratory flow when half of the forced vital capacity has been expelled — also sometimes called the forced expiratory flow at 50% of expiration (FEF_{50}) and sometimes calculated as the change in volume between 75% and 25% of the FVC divided by the time taken for this volume change (FEF_{25-75}). This parameter is largely independent of effort and reflects chiefly the severity of the obstruction in the smaller airways. It is an important measurement since it may well be abnormal when the PEF and even the FEV_1 are normal.

Other lung function tests
These are rarely needed, but can be useful when there is doubt about the diagnosis.

Flow-volume loop shows typical scalloping of expiratory flow with relatively normal inspiratory flow and is useful to differentiate upper airway obstruction.

Plethysmography shows increased airways resistance, increased total lung capacity and residual volume (hyperinflation), largely independent of patient effort.

Gas transfer: usually normal when corrected for lung volumes, but may be increased (helps to exclude emphysema in which it is reduced).

Lung function in young children

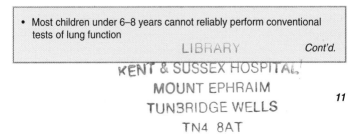

- Most children under 6–8 years cannot reliably perform conventional tests of lung function

Not every young child needs to perform lung function or bronchial challenge tests; these are most useful for those patients in whom the diagnosis of asthma is in doubt, or for those asthmatics in whom the severity of the disease is unclear from the history for whatever reason. In this context, bronchial hyperresponsiveness to methacholine is common to a number of chronic lung diseases besides asthma, including cystic fibrosis, but hyperreactivity to adenosine (like exercise in older patients) is highly specific for asthma.

Other investigations

Imaging
Chest radiographs are usually normal or show hyperinflation. In children, transient infiltrates in the middle lobe or lingula are not uncommon (and do not necessarily imply bacterial infection). A normal chest radiograph helps exclude other causes of airway obstruction. Bronchopulmonary aspergillosis may cause transient infiltrates and rare pulmonary eosinophilic syndromes may be associated with asthma.

Sinus radiographs are usually not informative (CT scan better).

CT scans are used only to document bronchiectasis and emphysema.

Allergen testing
Skin prick testing is used to document atopy and identify possible allergens. The most useful allergens are house dust mite,

grass pollen, cat fur and *Aspergillus fumigatus*. Histamine is used as a positive control, saline as a negative control.

RAST tests. Blood is tested for specific IgE; this is indicated only when skin testing is not possible (e.g. in severe eczema).

Blood tests

Eosinophilia (eosinophil count >300/dl or >2% of total leukocytes) is often absent. A very high count may indicate an eosinophilic syndrome (e.g. Churg–Strauss syndrome, polyarteritis nodosa, or bronchopulmonary aspergillosis).

Total IgE is not very useful. It is often elevated in children with gastrointestinal parasites.

Sputum examination

This characteristically shows eosinophilia.

Bronchial challenge studies

Histamine or methacholine inhalation challenge is occasionally used in diagnosis when lung function is normal but the history suggests asthma. Values of <8 mg/ml suggest airway hyperresponsiveness.

Exercise challenge is useful in children or young adults when there is doubt about the diagnosis. It is more specific but less sensitive than histamine or methacholine challenge.

Allergen challenge is not used routinely; it is usually a research tool.

Adenosine monophosphate (AMP) challenge may be more sensitive than histamine or methacholine challenge and is specific for asthma (currently a research tool).

Occupational challenge with a suspect chemical or occupational agent is confined to specialist centres.

Therapeutic challenge

Bronchodilator response. A short-acting inhaled β_2-agonist is used to demonstrate reversibility of lung function, or improvement in PEF at home (>15% improvement suggests asthma but a negative response does not exclude diagnosis).

Trial of steroids is used to differentiate chronic obstructive pulmonary disease (COPD) from chronic asthma. Oral prednisolone, 30–40 mg daily, is given for two weeks (in adults; appropriate lower dose in children), with twice daily recording of PEF and FEV_1 at the end of the trial. An increase of more than 15% indicates a diagnosis of asthma.

Bronchoscopy

This is not indicated routinely. Biopsy studies are used in research.

Differential diagnosis in adults

Asthma is usually easy to diagnose on the history and is confirmed by simple spirometry or peak flow monitoring. It is important to exclude some diseases in adults:

- Mechanical obstruction of airways (chest radiograph, bronchoscopy)
- COPD (history, lung function tests, trial of steroids)
- Heart failure (history, signs, chest radiograph)
- Pulmonary embolism (chest radiograph, ECG)
- Vasculitides, e.g. Churg–Strauss syndrome, polyarteritis nodosa, Wegener's granulomatosis (systemic symptoms and signs)
- Carcinoid syndrome with hepatic metastases (systemic symptoms, high urinary hydroxyindole acetic acid)

Differential diagnosis in children

There are special problems in diagnosing asthma in young children because the clinical features often differ from those in adults and older children. The commonest mode of presentation is recurrent episodes of respiratory distress characterized by coughing (invariably worse at night). The child almost always has completely symptom-free intervals, at least at first. Persistent symptoms, localized signs, failure to thrive, persistent radiological changes and other significant disease should raise the possibility of an alternative diagnosis.

Features suggestive of asthma in young children:
- Symptom-free intervals
- Nocturnal cough
- Coughing after exercise
- Coughing when laughing or crying
- Good response to correctly inhaled or nebulized bronchodilators
- Personal or family history of atopic disease
- Onset unrelated to respiratory syncytial virus (RSV) infection

Features suggestive of alternative diagnosis in young children:
- Failure to thrive (? cystic fibrosis, immunodeficiency)
- Absence of symptom-free intervals (? bronchiolitis obliterans, congenital anomaly)
- Sudden onset of persistent symptoms (? foreign body aspiration)
- Persistent URTI / otitis (? primary ciliary dyskinesia)
- Vomiting / recurrent pneumonia (? acid reflux, aspiration)
- Premature birth (? bronchopulmonary dysplasia)
- Onset in RS virus season (? post RSV bronchiolitis)

Principles of treatment

In several countries, guidelines for the management of asthma have been formulated by experts. These guidelines reconcile previously divergent approaches to treatment and are based on our current understanding of asthma and the mode of action of anti-asthma therapy.

In the guidelines the following points are emphasized:

- Educate patients to develop a partnership in asthma management
- Assess and monitor asthma severity with objective measurements of lung function
- Avoid or control asthma triggers
- Establish medication plans for chronic management
- Establish plans for managing exacerbations
- Provide regular follow-up care

Inherent in these guidelines is the need to recognize that the diagnosis is indeed asthma, and to evaluate the severity of the disease and the response to treatment. These objectives require the development of appropriate clinical and functional methods of evaluating the condition of the patient.

Recognition of asthma

Unless the patient, the family and the treating physician recognize that the patient is suffering from asthma, it is unlikely that he will receive correct treatment.

- Asthma in children is often misdiagnosed as bronchitis, wheezy bronchitis, or pneumonia
- Asthma in adults may be dismissed as COPD, chronic bronchitis, or emphysema

Asthmatics who are wrongly diagnosed are often treated with antibiotics, which are of no help, and fail to receive anti-asthma medication.

Clinical evaluation of severity

More information is obtained by taking a careful history from the asthmatic than by any other means, including physical examination and tests of lung function. In most patients, the important decisions on management are based largely on the severity of symptoms and their response to treatment. With some patients this is unreliable, either because the patient cannot give a clear history, for whatever reason, or because he does not feel the changes in severity of his airways obstruction.

In most cases, the clinical severity of asthma should be based on the following criteria, which reflect the amount of disturbance to the everyday life of the patient or his family. It is only practical to consider the 12 months before evaluation.

- The number of daytime attacks lasting more than 24 hours and needing extra medication
- The presence of completely symptom-free intervals lasting more than 4 weeks without medication
- The frequency of waking at night because of asthma symptoms
- The amount of absence from work or school because of asthma
- The ability of the patient to keep up with peers in normal physical activity
- The number and type of medications required on a regular daily basis
- The frequency of using extra relief medications on an 'as needed' basis
- The frequency of hospital admissions or Accident and Emergency Department attendances
- The frequency of any life-threatening episodes of acute asthma requiring intensive care

On the basis of this information the severity of asthma can be divided into broad groups, although the dividing line between them is somewhat subjective and will depend upon the symptom tolerance of the patient (Fig. 5).

Mild intermittent asthma

Patients have attacks requiring medication at infrequent intervals with long symptom-free periods. As a rule of thumb, the ratio of symptom-free to symptomatic days should be 10:1 or more. The patient should not lose more than the occasional day from work or school, should sleep undisturbed most nights and should be able to take normal physical activity, although extra medication may be needed if exercise-induced asthma is a problem.

Moderate perennial asthma

These patients are unwell more than they are well and will usually report symptoms daily or several times a week, unless

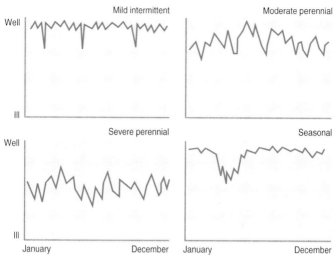

Figure 5

Diagrammatic representation of the common patterns of asthma. Asthma severity is arbitrarily represented on the vertical axis and one year on the horizontal axis.

they are receiving appropriate medication. Some absence from work or school is usual, nocturnal symptoms are common and exercise is often problematic. The asthma can usually be controlled with modest doses of medication on a regular basis.

Severe perennial asthma

These patients have daily or very frequent symptoms, are disturbed on most nights, cannot exercise normally and are prone to miss work or school. They require continuous medication in large doses to control their symptoms and need to attend their physician or hospital clinic at frequent intervals.

A distinction must be drawn between the overall clinical severity of asthma, as defined above, and the severity of individual exacerbations during the course of the disease. Patients with mild or moderate asthma may occasionally have a severe attack but this does not mean that they are severe asthmatics, as defined by the amount of disturbance to their everyday life.

In addition to the three groups described above, there are three special subgroups of asthma.

Seasonal asthma

Asthma may become much more troublesome or appear only during a particular time of the year because of a specific allergy causing a seasonal exacerbation, because of changes in weather conditions, or because of viral infections. Many children have much more asthma in the winter than in the summer. Patients with seasonal asthma may fall into the moderate or severe group during their bad season and the mild group during their good season. Medication should be adjusted accordingly.

Exercise-induced asthma (EIA)

Exercise is a potent stimulus for a short attack of bronchospasm in almost all asthmatics if they exercise hard enough (Fig. 6). There are some patients, mostly fit, young adolescents, who have little or no clinical asthma on a day-to-day basis but are severely handicapped by EIA when they take part in sports. Such patients can easily be dismissed as neurotic if the appropriate tests are not performed.

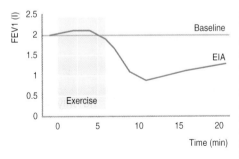

Figure 6
Typical exercise-induced asthma (EIA) in a child. During the six minutes of exercise there is a small improvement in lung function. Lung function begins to fall at the end of exercise and the attack of EIA reaches its greatest severity 5 minutes after the end of exercise.

Sudden life-threatening asthma

A few asthmatics suffer from infrequent but devastatingly severe attacks of asthma ('brittle' asthma), which often require admission to an intensive care unit and ventilatory support. It is not uncommon for the patient to be totally symptom-free in the intervals between attacks, with no need for medication. These patients present a very high-risk group and their management is problematical (see page 69).

Functional evaluation of severity

Spirometry

	Normal	Mild attack	Moderate attack	Severe attack
FEV_1 baseline	>80%	>70%	>60%	<60%
after bronchodilator	no change	>80%	>70%	no change
PEF baseline	>80%	>80%	>60%	<60%
after bronchodilator	no change	no change	>70%	no change
MEF baseline	>60%	>50%	>40%	<40%
after bronchodilator	no change	>60%	no change	no change

Table 1
Functional evaluation of severity by spirometry.

Ambulatory monitoring of PEF

Because of the realisation that the variability of lung function is the most important functional index of asthma severity and the best guide to asthma control, guidelines now recommend the use of home monitoring of lung function for patients with troublesome asthma (Fig. 7). At the present time, the only readily available and practical device for use on an ambulatory basis is the peak flow meter in one or other of its versions. Expensive spirometers for home use are also available and centralized monitoring of lung function using devices attached to the telephone is available in some countries. Exactly who should be monitored is a question of experience, in which the value of obtaining objective data must be weighed against the inconvenience and cost of performing the test and the possibility of inducing anxiety if the test is not always normal.

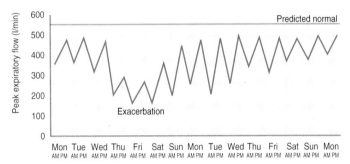

Figure 7
Peak flow chart showing exacerbation of asthma. The patient started a course of prednisolone on Thursday and gradually improved. Note the large diurnal variation in peak flow during the recovery period.

Monitoring not needed or impossible
- Young children
- Mild, intermittent asthma
- Seasonal asthma

Monitor continuously
- Severe perennial asthma with suboptimal lung function
- Sudden life-threatening asthma, even between attacks
- Patients involved in drug trials for asthma

Monitor in times of changing control
- Severe perennial asthma with usually good lung function
- Perennial asthma of uncertain severity
- Uncertain clinical severity or treatment requirements
- To demonstrate efficacy of inhaled/oral steroids and to confirm the diagnosis

Once home monitoring is recommended, the physician must explain to the patient exactly how to use the PEF meter and be certain that the patient can use it properly before leaving the clinic.

The correct technique is as follows:

- The test should be performed standing with the PEF meter held horizontally
- The patient should take a maximum inspiration and expel the breath as hard and fast as possible through the PEF meter (without coughing)
- At least 3 efforts should be made and the highest value recorded
- The test is usually performed twice daily (on waking and last thing at night, before taking any medications)
- Some recommend testing before and after a bronchodilator but this is hardly practical (or even desirable) on a day-to-day basis

Besides recording the best of the morning and evening PEF measurements the difference between morning and evening values (PEF variability) is important.

$$\frac{\text{evening PEF} - \text{morning PEF}}{(\text{evening PEF} + \text{morning PEF}) \times 0.5}$$

The evening PEF is usually higher than the morning value but it is only the size of the difference that is important. A PEF variability of >20% is considered to be abnormal.

The results of home PEF measurements are best recorded in an asthma diary, of which there are many simple variations; this is also the best place to record symptoms and drug consumption. It is important that information be obtained on the personal best value of PEF for each patient who never reaches the normal range. The time taken to determine this personal best will vary from patient to patient but sufficient time should be allowed to be sure that the current best value cannot be improved by better treatment.

Evaluation of the quality of asthma control

The goals of asthma management are:

- To abolish symptoms
- To restore normal or best possible airway function
- To reduce the risk of severe attacks
- To enable normal growth to occur in children
- To minimize absence from school or work
- In achieving these goals, to avoid side-effects of therapy

The evaluation of the quality of control of asthmatic symptoms whether by medication, avoidance of allergen exposure or any other method, is closely related to the evaluation of the severity of the disease by the clinical and/or physiological methods discussed above. In choosing treatment, the following criteria should be taken into account:

- The amount of disturbance to the everyday life of the patient and/or his family
- The response of the disease to the treatment prescribed
- The ability of the patient and/or the family to comply with the prescribed treatment

The continuing management of the patient requires a periodic review to determine whether the treatment plan prescribed in accordance with these principles achieves the goals of good control of asthma as defined above. This review may simply be infrequent clinic visits in the case of mild, well-controlled asthma or may require continuous recording of symptoms and PEF at home using an appropriate asthma diary in severe perennial asthma. Exactly what is needed in each case can only be determined by experience.

Treatment may need to be changed and this is best done in a controlled, step-wise fashion.

No change required
- Minimal symptoms but not necessarily totally asymptomatic
- No limitation of everyday activities, no loss of work or schooling
- Occasional need for extra bronchodilator medication
- PEF >80% predicted or personal best (if being recorded at home)
- PEF variability < 20% (if being recorded at home)
- No side-effects from medications

Increase medication
- Daily symptoms or frequent nocturnal asthma
- Reduced everyday activities or some loss of work or schooling
- Daily need for extra bronchodilator medication
- PEF < 80% predicted or personal best (if being recorded at home)
- PEF variability >20% (if being recorded at home)
- Side-effects from medications may require change in medication

Reduce medication
- No symptoms for at least 4 weeks
- No limitation of everyday activities, no loss of work or schooling
- No need for extra bronchodilator medication
- PEF >80% predicted (if being recorded at home)
- PEF variability < 20% (if being recorded at home)

After any change in treatment, the condition of the patient will need to be reviewed again periodically in case a further change in either direction is required.

Drug delivery

Asthma is a disease of the bronchial tree in which the airways are narrowed — the result of a combination of bronchospasm, inflammatory infiltration and secretion into the lumen. The most obvious and direct route for delivering drugs to the asthmatic airway is by inhalation and this route increases the local deposition while minimizing systemic effects. Fortunately, most of the medications needed to treat asthma can be delivered by inhalation. Other routes of medication, particularly oral and intravenous, may be more appropriate under some circumstances.

Inhaled route always recommended for
- β_2-agonists (except in some infants)
- Anticholinergics
- Cromones (sodium cromoglycate or nedocromil sodium)
- Corticosteroid prophylaxis (except in the severest unresponsive asthma)

Oral route recommended for
- β_2-agonists in infants with mild asthma
- Theophylline preparations for prophylaxis (always)

- Anti-leukotriene preparations for prophylaxis
- Corticosteroids for relief of acute attacks (short 'crash' course)
- Corticosteroid prophylaxis of severe asthma unresponsive to inhaled steroids
- Corticosteroid prophylaxis in small children or others unable to use inhalers

Intravenous route recommended for
- Corticosteroids for treatment of status asthmaticus (if unable to take oral steroids)
- Aminophylline if indicated for status asthmaticus
- β_2-agonists if indicated for status asthmaticus

Intramuscular route recommended for
- Depot corticosteroids for asthma uncontrolled by other methods (rarely indicated)

Drug delivery by the oral, intravenous or intramuscular routes poses no particular problem in asthma and follows normal clinical practice for delivering drugs by these routes. The indications for using different drugs and different routes are discussed more fully in other sections. Recommended doses are shown in the Appendix.

Administration of medications by inhalation

Given the central role of inhalation therapy for most asthma treatment it is important to understand the way in which different delivery systems work and how they should be used by the patient. Unless the physician understands the use of an inhaler device and can use it effectively, it is highly unlikely that his or her patients will do so. There are four basic systems currently available for delivering drugs by inhalation (Fig. 8).

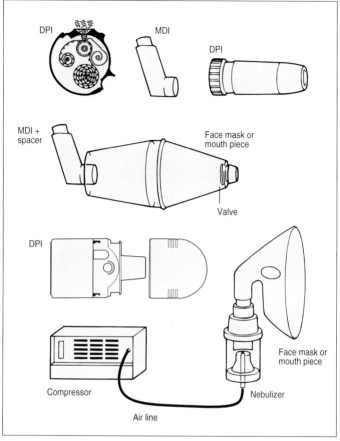

Figure 8

Various inhaler devices (not drawn to scale). Both spacer and nebulizer can be fitted with a mouthpiece for older and more co-operative patients, and with a face mask for younger or less co-operative patients. MDI= metered dose inhaler, DPI= dry powder inhaler.

Metered dose inhaler (MDI)

The MDI contains medication mixed with a chlorofluorocarbon (CFC) propellant (currently being replaced by a hydrofluoro-carbon, which has no effect on the ozone layer) and a controlled dose is emitted as a spray when the device is activated. It is a very convenient delivery system and MDIs are available for all common asthma medications, except theophylline preparations and anti-leukotrienes.

Advantages	Disadvantages	Correct technique
Small and portable	Good technique needed	Shake the inhaler
Cheap	Unsuitable for children < 5–6 years	Hold upright
Quick to use		Breathe out
	Unsuitable for the elderly, arthritic, etc.	Close lips around mouthpiece
	Cold jet may irritate throat	Fire device at start of slow inspiration
	Limited amount of drug delivered per puff	Inspire to total lung capacity
		Hold breath for 10 s
		Breath out

Metered dose inhaler with spacer (MDI+spacer)

Because many patients, both young and old, are unable to coordinate well enough to use an MDI correctly, various holding chambers (spacers) have been developed; these are placed between the MDI and the patient. The drug is inhaled from the chamber and coordination with the firing of the MDI is no longer important. Most spacers have some type of non-rebreathing valve. Some are large volume, some are much smaller, and there are spacers with face masks suitable for infants. The type of spacer used is probably of little importance in most cases.

Advantages	Disadvantages	Correct technique
Coordination unimportant	Bulky and inconvenient	Shake the inhaler
Can be used by all ages	Valves sometimes stick or become incompetent	Fix MDI upright in spacer
May reduce systemic absorption		Keep lips on mouth-piece or keep face mask tightly applied to face (infants)
May be effective even in severe asthma		Breathe in and out through spacer
Relatively inexpensive		Fire device while taking: 1–2 deep breaths (adults) 3–4 deep breaths (children)
		Be sure valve is operating
		Keep spacer clean and dry

When the treatment calls for two or more doses of medication, it is important that each dose be taken separately; it is not recommended that the MDI is activated more than once per inspiration or that the spacer is loaded with several doses.

Dry powder inhaler (DPI)
Several multi-dose devices have been developed from which the patient inhales a dry powder formulation of the drug. These

do not contain CFCs and since they are only activated by the inspiratory effort of the patient, coordination is not a problem, although the inhalation technique is still very important.

Advantages	Disadvantages	Correct technique
Coordination unimportant	Relatively expensive	Follow instruction for preparation of device
Can be used for most ages	Require rapid inspiration	Breathe out
Small and portable	Not suitable for children below the age of 5 years	Place lips firmly around mouthpiece
No CFCs		Breathe in rapidly and deeply
Multiple dry powder devices convenient, easy to operate		

The newer multidose types of powder inhalers are suitable for most patients, including those who would require a spacer in order to use an MDI. The lack of CFCs makes them environmentally attractive. They are not suitable for most children below the age of five to six years, or for patients who cannot inspire reasonably rapidly.

Nebulizer

Jet nebulizers produce a cloud of medication by passing a jet of compressed air over a solution of the drug. The less common *ultrasonic nebulizers* produce the cloud by dropping the solution into a plate which vibrates at high frequency. Preparations of bronchodilators, sodium cromoglycate and steroids (budesonide) are available for nebulization.

Advantages	Disadvantages	Correct technique
Coordination unimportant	Cumbersome equipment	Follow instruction for preparation of device
Can be used for all ages	Expensive	Normal breathing through mouthpiece or face mask
Effective in severe asthma	Noisy	
	Treatment takes a long time	Breathe continuously for at least 5–6 min
No CFCs	Disliked by some infants, loathed by others	

The actual dose of medication reaching the lungs from most devices is only about 10% of that delivered by the inhalation device, whether it be an MDI, DPI or nebulizer and, in many situations, it is even less. Much of the drug is impacted on the device itself; some particles are too large to reach the lungs and impact on the buccal mucosa, with the potential for systemic absorption. This is particularly important for inhaled steroids and there are some data to suggest that the use of a spacer reduces this unwanted effect. Even though the lung dose is relatively low, drug delivery by inhalation is usually highly effective if the correct technique is used.

Which inhalation device for which patient?

Infants and children up to about 5 years	MDI+spacer, Nebulizer
Children 5–9 years	MDI (?), MDI+spacer, DPI, Nebulizer
Competent older children/adults	MDI, DPI
Incompetent older children/adults	MDI+spacer, Nebulizer (?)

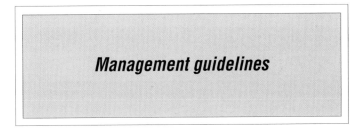

Management guidelines

Guidelines to asthma management have been adopted in many countries. Guidelines should be flexible and should change as new information becomes available.

A step-wise approach to management should be adopted (Fig. 9). Patients should start at the step a little above that most appro-

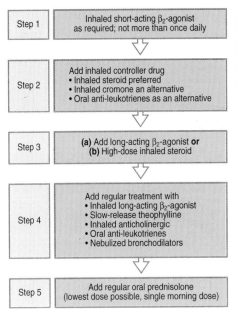

Step 1	Inhaled short-acting β_2-agonist as required; not more than once daily
Step 2	Add inhaled controller drug • Inhaled steroid preferred • Inhaled cromone an alternative • Oral anti-leukotrienes as an alternative
Step 3	(a) Add long-acting β_2-agonist **or** (b) High-dose inhaled steroid
Step 4	Add regular treatment with • Inhaled long-acting β_2-agonist • Slow-release theophylline • Inhaled anticholinergic • Oral anti-leukotrienes • Nebulized bronchodilators
Step 5	Add regular oral prednisolone (lowest dose possible, single morning dose)

Figure 9
Step-wise approach to asthma therapy. Start at a relatively high level and step down once control is achieved.

33

priate to the initial severity of asthma (see pages 17–21) and progress up or down to the next step according to when control cannot be achieved, providing medication is being used correctly. Once satisfactory control has been maintained for several months, treatment should be stepped down, so that the patient is maintained on the minimal treatment needed for optimal control. For recommended doses see the Appendix.

Avoidance

- Allergens: house dust mite, domestic pets, pollens. House dust mite avoidance using barrier methods is effective. Exclude domestic pets (especially cats) where possible
- Cigarette smoking (active and passive)
- Occupational causes of asthma should always be considered
- Beta-blockers (tablets and eye drops) in all patients
- Aspirin and non-steroidal anti-inflammatory drugs in patients with aspirin-sensitive asthma

Triggers such as exercise and cold air should not be avoided, but treatment should be adjusted to minimize symptoms.

Step 1: inhaled β_2-agonist as required

Use a short-acting β_2-agonist (e.g. salbutamol, terbutaline) as required for symptom relief. If it is required more than once daily, move to step 2 (but ensure patient has good inhaler technique). Concerns have been expressed about regular use and high doses of short-acting inhaled β_2-agonists.

Step 2: regular inhaled anti-inflammatory drugs

If the β_2-agonist inhaler is used more than once daily, or if nocturnal symptoms present, add an inhaled steroid (beclomethasone dipropionate, budesonide, fluticasone propionate bd). It is best to start with a higher dose (400 µg bd) and then reduce it once control is achieved.

As an alternative, cromones (sodium cromoglycate or nedocromil sodium) or antileukotrienes may be tried, but if control is not achieved in four weeks, start the patient on inhaled steroids.

Step 3: (a) add another controller

Add long-acting β_2-agonist (salmeterol 50 µg bd or formoterol 12 µg bd), low dose theophylline or anti-leukotriene to the current dose of inhaled steroid .

(b) high-dose inhaled steroids

If 3(a) is not effective increase inhaled steroids up to 2000 µg daily for adults or 1000 µg daily for children.

If using an MDI, use a large volume spacer; if using dry powder, always advise mouth washing.

Step 4: additional treatments

Add regular bronchodilators to high-dose inhaled steroids. A therapeutic trial of four weeks' therapy should be given sequentially.

- Inhaled salmeterol (50–100 µg bd) or formoterol (12–24 µg bd)
- Oral slow-release theophylline/aminophylline preparation
- Inhaled ipratropium/oxitropium bromide (tds/qds)
- Nebulized β_2-agonist (qds)
- Oral slow-release β_2-agonist (e.g. bambuterol 20 mg od)
- Oral anti-leukotrienes (e.g. montelukast 10 mg od)

Step 5: regular oral steroids

Add regular oral prednisolone in a single daily dose, using the minimal dose needed to maintain control. In a few patients, high regular doses may be needed; consider methotrexate, oral gold or cyclosporin A as a way to reduce the dose requirement. For children, it is preferable to give the oral steroids as a single dose on alternate mornings.

Step-down

Once control is achieved, treatment should be reviewed every 2–4 months initially. Step-wise reduction of treatment may be possible. In patients taking inhaled steroids, the dose should be reduced every 3–6 months to find the minimum required for control.

Before moving up from one step to the next, ensure that drugs are being taken correctly (check compliance and inhaler use).

When to refer to specialist clinic

- When there is doubt about diagnosis (e.g. failure to thrive in children; wheeze in elderly smoker; persistent cough; concomitant systemic symptoms, such as rash, arthritis, weight loss, proteinuria etc.)
- Patients with possible occupational asthma
- Patients whose asthma is difficult to control:
  brittle asthma
  continuing symptoms despite high-dose inhaled steroids (beyond Step 3)
  pregnant women whose asthma is worse
  patients whose asthma is interfering with their lifestyle
  patients with compliance and psychological problems
  patients who have recently been discharged from hospital
- Patients who require maintenance oral steroids

Asthma is by far the commonest troublesome chronic disease of childhood. It affects some 10–15% of school-age children and the incidence is steadily increasing. Almost all children with asthma are atopic and the clinical presentation is usually quite typical. A particular problem exists with asthma in infants and very young children because variable airways obstruction can also be due to acute viral bronchiolitis or its sequelae.

The wheezy infant

Wheezing lower respiratory tract illness is extremely common in the first 12–18 months of life and may affect almost all children in a closed community. The infant presents with tachypnoea, respiratory distress, prolonged expiration with late expiratory wheezing, and the chest radiograph shows hyperinflation. This picture may be due to acute infection with the respiratory syncytial virus (RSV), in which case it is usually a short self-limited illness (Table 2). However, a good proportion of such infants continue to have wheezing attacks for a number of months without new infections and without continuing to become typical asthmatic children later. On the other hand, about 20% of future asthmatic children have their first wheezing attacks in the first year of life. There may be some diagnostic clues but often it is impossible to be certain without pro-longed follow-up.

	Acute RSV bronchiolitis	Recurrent post-bronchiolitic wheezing	Infantile asthma
Epidemic	Yes — winter	No	No
Family asthma/atopy	Not especially	Not especially	Common
Response to anti-asthma therapy	Very poor	Rarely helpful	Sometimes helpful
Prognosis	Self-limited ($\approx$ 1 week)	Self-limited ($\approx$ 2 years)	Uncertain

Table 2
Differential diagnosis of lower respiratory tract illness in children.

No medications have been shown to alter the course of acute RSV bronchiolitis consistently and treatment is supportive, with added oxygen if necessary. It is almost irresistible to try anti-asthma medication for the recurrent post-bronchiolitic wheezy infant and occasionally they seem to respond. Unfortunately, many infant asthmatics also respond poorly to medication but as they get older, they develop the normal good responses of the asthmatic child. It is important to remember that chronic respiratory symptoms in infancy may be due to other serious diseases such as cystic fibrosis, recurrent aspiration, congenital anomalies or immunodeficiency disorders. *Beware of the chesty infant with failure to thrive.*

The asthmatic child

Children with asthma usually respond very well to treatment and almost all should be able to lead full normal lives, apart from the need for appropriate medication. The greatest problems with asthma in young children are:

- Failure to diagnose asthma in a child whose main symptom is cough, especially at night or after exertion
- Misdiagnosis of asthma as recurrent pneumonia because attacks are frequently precipitated by febrile (viral) illnesses
- Evaluation of disease activity usually depends on the impression of a third party
- Young children cannot use PEF meters reliably; older children often do not want to use them
- Need to give medications by inhalation which may present practical difficulties with inhalation devices and problems with timing of medication in children at school
- Anxiety of parents (and some doctors) about unwanted side-effects of treatment leading to sub-optimal treatment and limitation of everyday activities
- True adverse effects of the disease or its treatment on normal growth and development

It is very important to realize that true recurrent pneumonia is very rare in childhood and almost always indicates a serious underlying condition. Asthma should always be considered in a child with recurrent lower respiratory tract disease, especially when there are definite symptom-free intervals between attacks.

The management of asthma in children follows the general guidelines discussed previously, with the proviso that some paediatricians would prefer to try non-steroidal prophylaxis with sodium cromoglycate before starting treatment with inhaled steroids. The place of anti-leukotriene agents in the management of childhood asthma has not yet been determined.

The adolescent asthmatic — growing out of asthma

The large majority of children with asthma become symptom-free or very much better by the time they reach adulthood. This growing out of asthma may occur at any time during childhood and there are no reliable predictors of the duration of the disease in younger children. Some children who grow out of their asthma develop it again in later adult life.

Asthmatic children tend to have a rather late puberty and, on average, their puberty growth spurt is delayed by about 15 months in comparison with their non-asthmatic peers. This means that the asthmatic adolescent often appears to be smaller than his friends; this may be erroneously attributed to the medication he is taking especially if it includes cortico-steroids. Careful studies have shown that the delay in puberty is unrelated to the type of medication and that after passing through puberty, most asthmatics reach their normal expected height. Undoubtedly, daily systemic corticosteroid therapy for prolonged periods will stunt growth, but such treatment should never be required for the management of asthma in children.

Adolescents are more likely to engage in vigorous sports than other age groups and this may pose particular problems for the asthmatic, who may well be troubled by exercise-induced asthma (EIA). This EIA may be the only manifestation of asthma and should always be considered in an otherwise fit child with undue dyspnoea on exertion. Treatment of EIA by the use of an inhaled β_2-agonist before exercise is extremely successful and no child should be prevented from taking part in games because of asthma.

Relievers or bronchodilators give relatively rapid relief of symptoms and are believed to work predominantly by relaxation of airway smooth muscle (although several other effects on the airways may contribute to their anti-asthma effects). Relievers are believed to have no effect on the chronic inflammation of asthma.

Short-acting inhaled β_2-agonists

Mode of action

- β_2-receptors on airway smooth muscle: relaxation in large and small airways. Functional antagonists: reverse bronchoconstriction irrespective of cause
- Mast cell stabilizers (useful in protecting against allergen- and exercise-induced asthma)
- Experimentally reduce plasma exudation, reduce cholinergic reflexes
- Increase mucociliary clearance
- No effect on chronic inflammation in asthma

Recommended use

- Immediate relief of symptoms
- Should not be used regularly (tolerance of protective effects, possible increase in morbidity and mortality)
- Prevention of exercise-induced asthma

Side-effects

- Muscle tremor (direct effect on skeletal muscle β_2-receptors). More common in elderly patients
- Tachycardia (direct effect on atrial β_2-receptors, reflex effect from increased peripheral vasodilatation via β_2-receptors)
- Hypokalaemia (direct effect on skeletal muscle uptake of K^+ via β_2-receptors). Usually a small effect
- Restlessness
- Hypoxaemia (increased $\dot{V}/\dot{Q}$ mismatch due to pulmonary vasodilatation)
- Worsening of asthma control? (controversial: probably only applies to very high doses)

The choice of short-acting β_2-agonist is described in the Appendix.

Long-acting inhaled β_2-agonists

These include salmeterol and formoterol. Both give bronchodilatation and protection against bronchoconstriction for over 12 hours (Fig. 10).

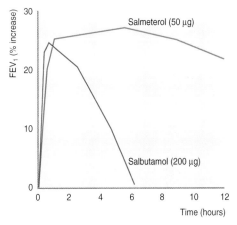

Figure 10
Bronchodilator effect of a long-acting inhaled β_2-agonist (salmeterol), compared with a short-acting β_2-agonist (salbutamol).

Recommended use

- As regular bronchodilators in patients taking moderate or high-dose inhaled steroids daily
- To gain asthma control in patients on low-dose inhaled steroids (400 µg daily) as an alternative to escalating the dose of inhaled steroids
- Useful in nocturnal asthma (single night-time dose sometimes useful)
- Prolonged protection against exercise-induced asthma
- No anti-inflammatory effect alone, therefore always use in combination with an inhaled steroid

Theophylline

This is classified as a bronchodilator, but relatively high doses are needed for airway smooth muscle relaxation. There is now increasing evidence that theophylline has anti-inflammatory or immunomodulatory effects at lower plasma concentrations (5–10 mg/l).

Mode of action

- Phosphodiesterase inhibition (increases cyclic AMP and cyclic GMP levels)
- Adenosine receptor antagonism (accounts for some side-effects, but little evidence that relevant for anti-asthma effects)
- Increased adrenaline secretion
- Prostaglandin inhibition
- Inhibition of calcium entry/release
- Inhibition of phosphoinositide hydrolysis
- Unknown: difficult to explain all of the anti-asthma effects of theophylline by above mechanisms, as many occur only at concentrations higher than those used therapeutically

Recommended use

- As additional bronchodilator in patients taking high-dose inhaled steroids
- Should be given as a trial of therapy (with PEF monitoring)
- Useful in combination with inhaled steroids for additional control of asthma as an alternative to high-dose inhaled steroids
- Useful in nocturnal asthma as single night-time dose
- Give either once or twice daily in dose to give plasma theophylline concentration of 5–10 mg/l

Side-effects

- Nausea and vomiting
- Headache
- Restlessness
- Gastro-oesophageal reflux
- Diuresis
- Cardiac arrhythmias (usually plasma concentration >20 mg/l)
- Epileptic seizures (usually plasma concentration >30 mg/l)

Clearance

Therapeutic effect is related to plasma concentration. Plasma concentration is affected by several factors that alter clearance, but with new recommendations on dose this is less likely to be a problem. If in doubt, measure the plasma concentration. Factors affecting theophylline clearance are listed below.

Increased clearance (increase dose)
- Enzyme induction (rifampicin, phenobarbitone, ethanol)
- Smoking (tobacco, marijuana)
- Childhood
- High-protein, low-carbohydrate diet
- Barbecued meat

Decreased clearance (decrease dose)
- Enzyme inhibition (cimetidine, erythromycin, ciprofloxacin, allopurinol, ketoconazole)
- Congestive heart failure
- Liver disease
- Pneumonia
- Viral infection and vaccination
- High-carbohydrate diet
- Old age

Anticholinergics

The most commonly used anticholinergics are ipratropium bromide (MDI or nebulizer qds) and oxitropium bromide (MDI tds/qds).

Mode of action

These drugs are muscarinic receptor antagonists, which inhibit cholinergic reflex bronchoconstriction and reduce vagal cholinergic tone.

Recommended use

- Additional bronchodilator in patients taking high-dose inhaled steroids. Always give trial of therapy (most useful in the elderly and in infants as first-line bronchodilator)
- Bronchodilator of choice in patients with COPD (in which vagal tone is a major reversible component)
- As an addition to nebulization of β_2-agonist in management of acute severe asthma

Side-effects

- Paradoxical bronchoconstriction (usually due to additives in nebulizer solution)
- Glaucoma (with nebulized drug when used without mouthpiece)
- Bitter taste
- Systemic effects such as dry mouth, urinary retention, constipation: very rare

Controllers

The term controller implies treatment that suppresses the underlying inflammatory process in asthmatic airways. The previously used term, anti-inflammatory treatment, is unsatisfactory as there are several types of inflammation. Thus, β_2-agonists are anti-inflammatory in the sense that they inhibit the release of inflammatory mediators from mast cells, yet they do not reduce the chronic inflammation in asthmatic airways (as measured in bronchial biopsies). Corticosteroids are the only drugs that have been shown to significantly reduce the inflammation in asthmatic airways.

Inhaled corticosteroids

Inhaled steroids are now introduced at a much earlier stage in treatment and are the controllers of choice in the management of most adult patients with asthma. Many paediatricians still prefer to start treatment with sodium cromoglycate if it is effective.

Mode of action

- Bind to cytosolic glucocorticoid receptors that regulate the expression of multiple genes (Fig. 11)
- Inhibit the synthesis of multiple cytokines involved in asthmatic inflammation, particularly IL-5, thus reducing eosinophilic infiltration into airways
- Inhibit the production of other inflammatory mediators, such as leukotrienes and prostaglandins
- Inhibit plasma exudation and mucus secretion
- Increase expression of airway β_2-receptors and prevent desensitization of β_2-receptors
- Prevent tissue remodelling?

Clinical efficacy

- Effective in virtually all patients, irrespective of age or severity of asthma
- Reduce asthma symptoms
- Improve lung function
- Reduce airway hyperresponsiveness (though not usually back to normal). Improvement occurs slowly over several months
- Reduce frequency of asthma attacks and hospital admissions
- Reduce asthma mortality?
- Prevent irreversible airway narrowing?
- Effects reverse when stopped (i.e. suppress inflammation, but do not cure underlying cause)

Recommended use

Doses given in the text refer to beclomethasone dipropionate (BDP) and the doses of the more modern fluticasone propionate (twice as potent) or budesonide via a dry powder inhaler (twice as much deposited in airways) will normally be half these:

- Use in any patient taking a short-acting inhaled β_2-agonist more than once daily
- Start at relatively high dose (800–1200 μg daily in adults) to establish effective control of asthma rapidly, then reduce to minimal dose needed over 6 months
- Use twice daily on a regular basis (at low doses, once daily may suffice). When asthma is unstable qds administration is preferable
- Increase to a maximal dose of 2000 μg daily (in adults) or 1000 μg daily (in children). Above these doses, systemic effects occur more frequently
- Budesonide and fluticasone preferable to beclomethasone dipropionate when larger doses are needed: less systemic effects
- Use a large volume spacer or mouth washing when high doses needed

The choice of inhaled steroid is described in the Appendix.

The dose equivalence of different inhaled steroids is influenced by the delivery systems used.

Side-effects
Side-effects are the major issue in the long-term use of inhaled steroids. They are mainly related to the inhaled dose, but some patients appear to have a greater susceptibility.

Local side-effects

- Due to deposition of inhaled steroid in the oropharynx
- Markedly reduced by use of a large volume spacer with an MDI, or mouth washing with a dry powder inhaler
- Hoarseness (dysphonia): commonest side-effect (occurs in up to 40% of patients taking high doses)
- Oropharyngeal candidiasis: occurs in approximately 5% of patients
- Throat irritation and cough (most likely to be due to additives in MDI; rarely occur with dry powder inhalers)

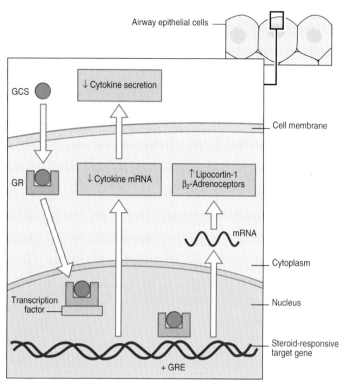

Figure 11

Molecular mechanisms of action of steroids in asthma. The glucocorticosteroid (GCS) binds to a glucocorticoid receptor (GR) in the cytoplasm of the target cell. The activated GR then moves into the nucleus, where it binds to a specific DNA-binding site (glucocorticoid response element, GRE) on the promoter region of target genes. This may increase transcription resulting in increased synthesis of protein (eg, β_2-receptors, lipocortin-1). Alternatively, GR binds to a transcription factor (DNA binding protein) that switches on inflammatory genes and thus prevents transcription, with reduced synthesis of inflammatory proteins such as cytokines.

Systemic side-effects

Systemic side-effects are due to absorption of inhaled steroids from the gastrointestinal tract and the respiratory tract (Fig. 12).

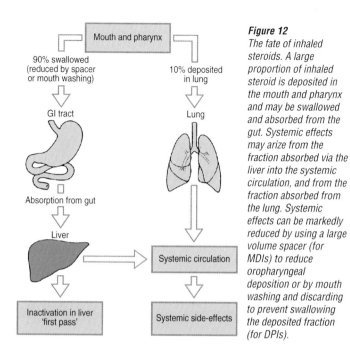

Figure 12
The fate of inhaled steroids. A large proportion of inhaled steroid is deposited in the mouth and pharynx and may be swallowed and absorbed from the gut. Systemic effects may arize from the fraction absorbed via the liver into the systemic circulation, and from the fraction absorbed from the lung. Systemic effects can be markedly reduced by using a large volume spacer (for MDIs) to reduce oropharyngeal deposition or by mouth washing and discarding to prevent swallowing the deposited fraction (for DPIs).

The gastrointestinal fraction is markedly reduced by a large volume spacer or mouth washing.

There are many reports of systemic side-effects after inhaled steroids but these are often difficult to interpret as the patients had also received courses of systemic steroids. There are now several controlled trials documenting systemic effects of inhaled steroids using sensitive indices, such as metabolic markers of bone metabolism (plasma osteocalcin, urinary pyridinium cross-links), short-term growth (knemometry) and suppression of adrenal function. Whether a small inhibitory effect in a very sensitive test is clinically relevant in terms of statural growth in children, or bone density and risk of osteoporosis in adults is not yet certain. The described side-effects include:

- Adrenal suppression
- Easy bruising
- Skin thinning
- Increased bone turnover, osteoporosis?
- Cataracts
- Stunted growth in children?
- Behavioural disturbances?

Most studies have shown no clinically relevant systemic effects at daily doses of less than 400 µg in children or less than 800 µg in adults.

Cromones

Cromones include sodium cromoglycate (qds via MDI, Spinhaler or nebulizer) and nedocromil sodium (tds/qds via MDI).

Mode of action

- Mast cell stabilization (but other drugs with mast cell stabilising properties are not effective in asthma)
- Inhibit sensory nerve activation
- Inhibitory effect on several types of inflammatory cell (eosinophils, macrophages, neutrophils) in vitro
- Inhibit indirect bronchial challenges (allergen, exercise, cold air, SO_2, bradykinin), but no effect on direct challenges (histamine, methacholine)
- No convincing evidence for an anti-inflammatory effect in asthmatic patients

Clinical efficacy

- Reduce asthma symptoms in some patients with mild-to-moderate asthma, especially in children. No obvious clinical indicators of patients who respond
- Effective in preventing allergen- and exercise-induced symptoms if taken immediately prior to trigger (but not as effective as a β_2-agonist)
- May be given as nebulized form (20 mg qds) in infants
- Should be taken 4 times daily — short duration of action
- Less effective than inhaled steroids. Used by some in children as a trial of therapy before starting inhaled steroids. Little used in adults
- No evidence for additive effect with steroids and little evidence for useful steroid-sparing effect

Side-effects

- Extremely rare with cromoglycate
- Angioneurotic oedema (very rare)
- Coughing immediately after administration (prevented by a β_2-agonist)
- Bitter taste (nedocromil only). Now available in menthol aerosols to mask taste
- Burning sensation (nedocromil only): due to activation of thermoreceptors

Anti-leukotrienes

Anti-leukotrienes include drugs that block leukotriene receptors (leukotriene antagonists, such as zafirlukast and montelukast) and drugs that inhibit the synthesis of leukotrienes (5-lipoxygenase inhibitors, such as zileuton). This is the first new class of drug introduced into asthma therapy for 25 years and these drugs are now becoming available in several countries.

Mode of action

- Leukotriene antagonists block the effects of leukotriene D_4 in airways and thus prevent all the bronchoconstrictor and other airway actions of leukotrienes that are generated in asthma
- 5-Lipoxygenase inhibitors inhibit the synthesis of all leukotrienes and have similar clinical effects to leukotriene antagonists
- There is an inhibitory effect in bronchoconstriction induced by exercise, hyperventilation and allergen (50–70% inhibition) and by aspirin in aspirin-sensitive asthmatics (100% inhibition)
- There is some evidence for an anti-inflammatory effect, although this is not as marked as with steroids

Clinical efficacy

- There is a small and variable bronchodilator effect, suggesting resting leukotriene production in asthma
- There is improvement in asthma symptoms, lung function and the need for rescue inhaled β_2-agonsts in clinical trials, but the degree of improvement is not as great as expected with inhaled steroids
- Some patients (e.g. aspirin-sensitive asthmatics) show an extremely good response, whereas others do not show any improvement.
- Anti-leukotrienes are effective as oral therapy and this may improve compliance with long-term therapy
- They may be tried in mild asthma as an initial controller medication
- They may be added to low or high doses of inhaled steroids to achieve better control
- In all cases a trial of therapy (4 weeks) should be given to document objective improvement in asthma control before continuing as regular therapy

Side-effects

- No class-specific side-effects have yet been reported
- For some drugs a proportion of patients develop abnormalities in liver function, so that liver function tests need to be checked on a regular basis

Oral steroids

Regular oral steroids are indicated only in the most severe asthmatic patients who cannot be controlled with high-dose inhaled steroids and additional regular bronchodilators: short courses of oral steroids are commonly used to treat exacerbations of asthma.

The oral steroid of choice is *prednisolone* given as a single daily dose (usually in the morning), as this steroid has the least systemic effects. Prednisolone is prefered to prednisone, which has to be converted to prednisolone in the liver. Deflazacort is a new oral steroid that is claimed to have less effect on bone metabolism, but it is more expensive than other oral steroids. In children it is preferable to give alternate morning doses if possible to reduce systemic side-effects. This may be the only effective therapy in very young children unable to use inhaled steroids.

Triamcinolone acetonide injections are slow-release preparations of systemic steroids. Some patients who have poor compliance may be helped by this treatment, which is given once monthly. There is a risk of developing proximal myopathy with this fluorinated steroid.

Short courses of oral steroids

- Indicated for exacerbations of asthma (see Acute exacerbations, page 63)
- Course should normally last 5–10 days
- Use enteric coated (EC) tablets if gastrointestinal disturbance

Maintenance oral steroids

- Use minimum dose needed to control asthma
- Change doses slowly (adrenal suppression)
- Issue patient with a steroid card (and Medic-alert bracelet should be worn if possible)
- Increase dose if severe infection, major trauma, surgery, dental treatment

Side-effects

- Adrenal suppression
- Cushingoid appearance
- Osteoporosis, spontaneous fractures
- Stunted growth
- Easy bruising
- Gastrointestinal symptoms
- Diabetes
- Hypertension
- Cataracts (post-capsular)
- Mental disturbance (euphoria, depression, mania)
- Increased weight (fluid retention and increased appetite)

Steroid-sparing therapies

In some patients who require maintenance oral steroids, serious side-effects such as osteoporosis, gastric ulceration, or diabetes, are an indication for introduction of a steroid-sparing therapy. These treatments usually have a high frequency of side-effects themselves and are therefore indicated only if the side-effects of oral steroids are a problem. In controlled trials of asthma, these therapies have been shown to reduce prednisolone requirements by 5–10 mg daily, but are more effective in some patients than others.

Methotrexate

- Use low dose (15 mg weekly, either orally or intra-muscularly)
- Side-effects include nausea and vomiting (common; less if initial dose reduced), hepatic fibrosis, blood dyscrasias, opportunistic infections

Gold

- Small steroid-sparing effect
- Side-effects include renal damage (nephrotic syndrome), hepatic dysfunction

Cyclosporin A

- Active against CD4$^+$ (helper) T-cells
- Has steroid-sparing effects in some patients in low dose (5 mg/kg daily)
- Side-effects include renal damage, hepatic dysfunction
- Monitor creatinine, liver function and blood pressure (check blood level)
- Only continue if clear objective benefit obtained

Other therapies

Ketotifen
- Antihistamine with sedative effects
- Controlled trials show little, if any, beneficial effect in children or adults

Antihistamines
- Not clinically useful in controlling asthma symptoms
- Non-sedative antihistamines (terfenadine, astemizole, loratadine) useful for concomitant rhinitis

Non-steroidal anti-inflammatory drugs
- No beneficial effect and may cause exacerbation of symptoms in patients with aspirin-sensitive asthma

Mucolytics
- No proven benefit in asthma treatment

Immunotherapy
- Of little proven value in most asthmatics with some risk of side-effects. In highly selected patients with unavoidable specific allergy of clinical relevance immunotherapy may be tried by a specialist in this form of therapy. Side-effects (local reactions and anaphylaxis) outweigh any benefit. May be indicated in highly selected patients

Calcium antagonists
- No beneficial effect in clinical asthma
- Useful in treating hypertension and ischaemic heart disease (as β-blockers absolutely contraindicated)

Alpha-blockers
- No proven value in treatment of asthma symptoms
- Useful as additional treatment for hypertension

Acute exacerbations

Every year, patients with asthma die of their disease and from analyses of the circumstances it appears that the large majority (over 80%) of such deaths are avoidable, and result either from incompetent management of acute exacerbations, or from negligence on the part of the patient or his family. The correct management of acute exacerbations of asthma (Fig. 13) is essential if this mortality is to be avoided and depends upon:

For ambulatory patients
- Correct interpretations of warning symptoms at home
- Correct treatment at home
- Recognition when hospital treatment is needed

For patients coming to hospital
- Correct evaluation in Accident and Emergency Department
- Correct treatment in Accident and Emergency Department
- Recognition when transfer to intensive care is needed
- Correct timing of discharge from hospital

For all patients
- Correct follow-up and modification of treatment

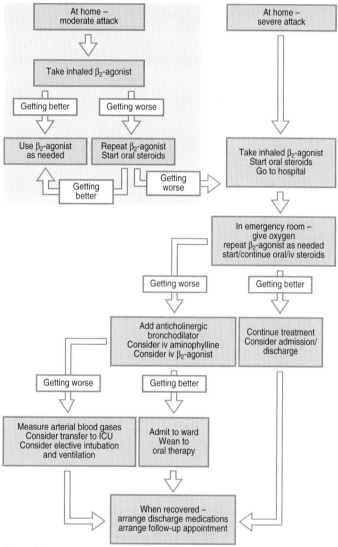

Figure 13
Algorithm for the management of acute asthma, the details of which are amplified in the text. The management shown surrounded by the tinted area in the upper left corner relates to moderate acute asthma not requiring hospitalisation unless it is unresponsive to treatment at home.

Symptoms of acute asthma

The symptoms of acute asthma are shown in Table 3. If the attack is severe but not life-threatening use the recommended ambulatory treatment.

	Adult	Child
Too breathless to talk normally	Yes	Yes
Tachypnoea	>25/min	>50/min
Tachycardia	>110/min	>140/min
PEF (if available)	< 50% predicted or personal best	rarely available

Table 3
Symptoms of acute asthma.

Ambulatory treatment for non-life-threatening attack

For doses of medications, see the Appendix.

Step 1
- Nebulized β_2-agonist bronchodilator if nebulizer available or
- MDI + spacer β_2-agonist (MDI alone if spacer unavailable)

Step 2
- Feeling better — repeat bronchodilator every 2–4 hours until back to usual state
- No better — repeat step 1 after 20 minutes and if still no better, move to

Step 3
- Start oral steroids as 7–10 day short course and repeat bronchodilator after 20 min. An anticholinergic may be added
- If no better consider going straight to hospital or call an ambulance

Potentially life-threatening attack in adults or children

Patients who present with the following:

- cyanosis of lips or tongue
- confusion, coma or agitation
- exhaustion, feeble respiratory effort
- PEF (if available) < 33% predicted or best

Should be given the recommended treatment and taken straight to hospital.

Treatment at home and on way to hospital

Oxygen if available
Nebulized β_2-agonist, if nebulizer available, or
MDI + spacer β_2-agonist (MDI alone if spacer unavailable)
Add inhaled anticholinergic if available
First dose of oral prednisolone.

Evaluation in Accident and Emergency Department — as above, plus

History of present illness and all medications taken in past 24 hours
Quick, relevant physical examination
Peak flow measurement if possible
Pulsus paradoxus suggests severe asthma
Bradycardia, hypotension suggest severe asthma
Pulse oximetry — saturation < 90% on room air suggests severe asthma
Urgent chest radiograph if pneumothorax suspected but don't delay treatment
Arterial blood gas analysis if asthma thought to be severe

Treatment in Accident and Emergency Department

Step 1
- Oxygen by face mask or nasal cannulae to keep saturation >95%
- Nebulized β_2-agonist (some prefer to use MDI + spacer β_2-agonist)
- Consider combining with nebulized ipratropium bromide (additional bronchodilator effect without increase in β_2-agonist side-effects)
  plus
- Oral prednisolone or
- Methylprednisolone/ hydrocortisone intravenously if oral route unsuitable

If the patient improves, progress to
Step 2a
- Oxygen as needed
- Repeat bronchodilator every 2–4 hours
- Oral/iv corticosteroids every 6 hours
- Monitor PEF, heart rate, respiratory rate and saturation

Step 2b
- Stop intravenous therapy
- Regular inhaled bronchodilators
- Oral corticosteroids
- Consider discharge and changes in regular medication

If the patient does not improve after step 1, progress to
Step 3a
- Add nebulized anticholinergic if not already being used
- Nebulized bronchodilators every 20 min
- Consider iv aminophylline (only maintenance dose if patient takes theophylline preparations at home)
- Consider iv β_2-agonist
- Repeat blood gas measurement
- Measure theophylline level if aminophylline is being used
- Measure electrolytes and glucose
- Beware of inappropriate ADH secretion — do not overload with fluids

Consider moving the patient to intensive care if
- Becoming comatose
- Becoming tired with weak respiratory effort
- Arterial PO_2 < 60 mmHg (< 8 kPa) or saturation < 90% on >60% inspired O_2
- Arterial PCO_2 > 45 mmHg (>6 kPa)

Remember that elective intubation and ventilation is always better than an emergency procedure. Never give sedatives unless the patient is intubated and ventilated. When the patient starts improving with or without a period of ventilation, continue as in steps 2a and 3a.

Discharge and follow-up

Criteria for discharge from hospital

- Symptom-free or return to usual ambulatory condition
- Good air entry and wheeze-free on examination
- PEF >75% predicted or personal best
- Saturation >92% breathing room air
- Full understanding of medications to be taken
- Ability to use any prescribed inhaler device correctly
- Discharge medications being taken correctly while still in hospital
- Adequately supportive home conditions

Discharge medications should include:
- Steadily reducing course of oral corticosteroids over about 1 week
- Regular inhaled bronchodilators until completely symptom-free, then as needed
- Increased dose of inhaled corticosteroids for 2–3 weeks if taken before admission
- Consider starting prophylaxis if not used before admission

Discharge arrangements should include:
- Adequate discharge summary for family physician
- Follow-up appointment for respiratory out-patient clinic within 1–2 weeks
- Written self management 'action plan' (revised if necessary)
- Asthma symptom diary if considered necessary
- PEF meter to use regularly at home if considered necessary
- Attempt to avoid contact with any overt asthma-precipitating factors

Special considerations

There are a number of situations in which the behaviour of asthma differs from the common patterns of the disease. Failure to recognize these variants for what they are may lead to misdiagnosis and mismanagement.

Exercise-induced asthma (EIA)

While most asthmatics will develop a short attack of asthma as a result of physical exercise, this is commonest in fit adolescents and young adults who take part in vigorous sports. In these patients it may be the only troublesome manifestation of the disease. The problem can be avoided or dealt with by recommending appropriate types of exercise and appropriate medication. Asthmatics should be encouraged to take part in normal physical activities.

EIA is due to the hyperventilation of exercise, which causes cooling and drying of the airway surface. This in turn may lead to the release of bronchoconstricting mediators from mast cells and the activation of sensory nerves, resulting in bronchoconstriction.

The conditions most likely to cause an attack of EIA are:
- 6–8 minutes of continuous hard exercise breathing cool or dry air
- Exercise during the allergy season in allergic asthmatics
- Failure to take appropriate medication

The conditions least likely to cause an attack of EIA are:
- Intermittent exercise, e.g. many team games
- Swimming or other exercise breathing warm humid air
- Premedication with an inhaled β_2-agonist bronchodilator

Nocturnal asthma

Nearly all asthmatics have worse asthma during the night than by day. This is often manifest in children by waking at night, coughing or wheezing, and in adults by waking early in the morning with chest tightness. This diurnal variation in asthma severity is very common and is a manifestation of airway hyperresponsiveness (Fig. 14).

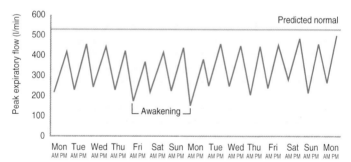

Figure 14
Peak flow record showing the typical diurnal variation in peak flow associated with nocturnal asthma. This patient awoke on two occasions during the period of recording.

Although the mechanism of nocturnal asthma is not completely understood, it may be related to circadian changes in circulating adrenaline and cortisol and vagal cholinergic tone. There is also evidence that airway inflammation and airway hyperresponsiveness increase at night.

The best method of dealing with this problem is to give the patient effective anti-inflammatory medication throughout the 24 hours. If symptoms persist add either a long-acting inhaled β_2-agonist at night, or a slow-release theophylline preparation.

Aspirin- and NSAID-sensitive asthma

A small proportion of asthmatics, almost always adults with relatively late-onset non-atopic asthma, are sensitive to aspirin and other non-steroidal anti-inflammatory drugs (NSAIDs). These patients commonly also have nasal polyps and perennial rhinitis. The ingestion of aspirin or other NSAID initially causes vasomotor rhinitis but later the patient responds to ingestion by developing an attack of asthma which may be very severe and even life-threatening.

The mechanism involves increased production of bronchoconstricting leukotrienes by blockade of the cyclo-oxygenase pathway.

It is important to enquire about the possible association of asthma attacks and NSAID ingestion, especially in adult-onset asthma, because these drugs are best avoided for life. Most such patients can tolerate paracetamol. Desensitization may be possible if NSAID therapy is essential, but this requires expert supervision.

Anti-leukotrienes may be the treatment of choice for these patients.

Pregnancy

The effect of pregnancy on the woman with asthma is uncertain since in some the disease becomes easier to control, in some it becomes more difficult, and in others there is no change; there are no means of predicting the response of the individual.

None of the important drugs used to treat asthma, such as the β_2-agonists, sodium cromoglycate and inhaled steroids, have been shown to have any adverse effect on the fetus or mother, while hypoxia is certainly bad for both. Every effort should be made to control asthma symptoms and maintain near normal lung function by the use of conventional medications, increasing the dose of inhaled steroids if necessary. Oral steroids can also be safely used when needed. On the whole, it is best to avoid adrenaline but this drug is rarely indicated.

It is important to stop mothers smoking, as there is good evidence that smoking increases the risk of developing asthma in infants. Smoking also causes fetal growth retardation, as well as adversely affecting the mother's asthma.

Gastro-oesophageal reflux (GR)

GR is not uncommon in infancy, even in the absence of any neurological disturbance, and the clinical picture of micro-aspiration may mimic asthma, with short episodes of reversible airways obstruction. This is distinct from massive aspiration, which causes pneumonia.

There is considerable debate about the importance of GR in older asthmatics, since some patients with particularly resistant asthma seem to benefit from antireflux medication or even surgery. Bronchodilators (β_2-agonists and theophylline) may increase acid reflux, and inhaled medication is preferred in patients with symptoms. A trial of effective antireflux therapy is indicated if there are symptoms (proton pump inhibitors, such as omeprazole, are more effective than H_2-antagonists, such as ranitidine).

Occupational asthma

Occupational asthma is a very specialized field and full of pitfalls for those unaware of the important clinical and medicolegal ramifications. There is no doubt that some agents can cause asthma to develop in some individuals who have never before had the disease, and can make asthma worse in those who have. The latency period may be months or even years after first exposure, which makes diagnosis all the more difficult. Typically, the asthma will steadily deteriorate during the working week, only to get better when exposure ceases at the weekend or when on holiday. The symptomatic complaints should be checked by daily PEF measurement. When there appears to be a true link to a particular agent, a challenge test should be performed under controlled laboratory conditions that mimic the working conditions as closely as possible. The best treatment is to avoid the offending substance but the patient may also require regular anti-asthma medication. It is not uncommon for the asthma to persist even after leaving the workplace.

Brittle 'catastrophic' asthma

One of the less common types of asthma is that in which the patient suffers from sudden, devastatingly severe attacks, which may occur against a background of apparently normal health. These patients are at risk from dying suddenly and should be treated with the utmost care. They should always carry emergency supplies of medications plus the necessary equipment to effectively administer a high dose of β_2-agonist (MDI with or without spacer), and a supply of oral corticosteroids which should be swallowed at the first sign of deterioration. Some patients may need to carry self-injectable adrenaline if the attacks develop so rapidly or are so severe that inhaled medication is of no value. The patient should always carry written instructions about emergency treatment and, if possible, a Medic-Alert bracelet, in case he is unable to administer medications himself. Some patients with frequent marked variations in PEF may be helped by subcutaneous β_2-agonist infusions (via insulin pump). Many would place this type of patient on continuous anti-inflammatory treatment even though their attacks are often infrequent.

Steroid-resistant asthma

Some asthmatics, mostly adults but occasionally children or adolescents, appear to be resistant to all forms of conventional medication, including corticosteroid therapy. In such patients, it is important to be sure that they do indeed have asthma and not some other condition such as cystic fibrosis, GR, bronchiolitis obliterans or emphysema, and it is equally important to be sure that they are taking their prescribed medications correctly and regularly. In the majority of such patients there will be a simple technical reason to explain the poor response, such as poor inhaler technique, poor compliance with treatment, or emotional disturbance. All apparently resistant patients should be given a trial of oral corticosteroids (prednisolone 40–60 mg daily for 2 weeks in adults) which also provides the opportunity to check compliance by measurement of diurnal cortisol levels and plasma prednisolone levels (when available). Sometimes these patients may respond to parenteral depot steroid preparations, such as triamcinolone acetonide and this may also serve as a check on patient compliance with treatment.

True steroid resistance is very rare and appears to be due to an abnormality in the interaction between the glucocorticoid receptor and DNA.

A more common occurrence is relative resistance, when patients require high doses of oral steroid to control their asthma. This may be helped by steroid-sparing therapies (methotrexate, oral gold, cyclosporin A) and by reducing the dose of inhaled β_2-agonists. Long-acting inhaled β_2-agonists and theophylline may be helpful in these patients; anti-leukotrienes may also be beneficial.

Practical matters

Patient education and doctor–patient relationships

The successful management of asthma depends to a very large degree on providing the patient with a good understanding of the nature of asthma and its treatment. The physician must take time to explain this to the patient in terms that he (or the parents of a small child) can understand, and the message must be reinforced at subsequent visits. There are a number of important points that need to be made:

- There is no cure for asthma but there is excellent treatment which can allow virtually all asthmatics to lead normal lives. There may be long-term or even permanent remissions of the disease, especially in children
- Asthma is rarely fatal but in those cases where it is, there has almost always been inadequate treatment or failure to comply with medical advice
- Far more patients die because they do not get corticosteroid therapy than the reverse. In conventional doses, corticosteroids are not harmful to either children or adults and they form the mainstay of the treatment of serious chronic asthma at all ages
- Compliance with treatment is essential and the major causes of inadequate control of asthma and consequent suffering are the 3 big Fs:
  - Failure to take prescribed medications regularly
  - Failure to take the prescribed dose
  - Failure to use inhalers properly
- The physician should make every attempt to verify compliance with treatment at each visit and should always check on inhaler technique and the functioning of spacer devices

- Alternative medicine such as acupuncture, homoeopathy and reflexology have little or no proven value in treating asthma and must never be used as a substitute for conventional medication, except in those with minimal disease. If the patient so desires, they may be added to conventional therapy
- Consultation with alternative medicine practitioners by the patient with troublesome asthma almost always means that the patient has not been given adequate information and has not been treated correctly by his conventional practitioner
- Some types of conventional therapy (e.g. antihistamines such as ketotifen, cromoglycate in steroid-dependent patients and immuno-therapy) add little, if anything, to the management of patients with significant asthma and should be stopped so that the patient needs to take only the minimum number of drugs to control his symptoms
  The simpler the regimen, the more likely is patient compliance and successful control of asthma

Ancillary devices to aid management

Given the fact that the management of asthma is ambulatory for most patients almost all of the time, the physician often needs objective information on the condition of the patient while engaged in normal activities. The patient also needs to know what to do about his treatment without consulting the physician at every turn. A number of ancillary devices have been developed for these purposes.

Diary cards

The simplest and possibly the most useful device is a daily record of symptoms and drug consumption. The patient is asked to fill in a card each day to record the intensity of nocturnal and daytime symptoms and the number of doses of all medications consumed. These diaries are particularly useful when evaluating a new patient, or when changing treatment regimens. They also provide a useful check on patient compliance (Fig. 15).

Year 1996 Month Jan	Day		1	2	3	4	5	6
Nighttime or early morning cough/wheeze	None − 0 Mild − 1 Moderate − 2 Severe − 3		0	1	2	1	0	1
Daytime cough/wheeze	None − 0 Mild − 1 Moderate − 2 Severe − 3		0	0	2	2	1	0
Limitation of activity/exercise	None − 0 Mild − 1 Moderate − 2 Severe − 3		0	0	1	1	0	0
Preventer medications Name (strength) *Pulmicort (200)*	Doses/day taken		4	4	4	3	4	4
Reliever medications Name (strength) *Ventolin (100)*	Doses/day taken		0	1	3	2	2	1
Morning PEF Evening PEF	Best of 3 Best of 3		420 450	410 460	350 400	300 310	350 410	400 420
Comments								

Figure 15
Diary for recording asthma symptoms, peak flow and medications, suitable for both children and adults.

Peak flow recording

Originally, PEF recording was introduced as an addendum to the diary score, to provide more objective data to go along with the subjective observations of the patient. In recent years, great emphasis has been placed on the continuous use of PEF meters at home by all chronic asthmatics, with treatment guidelines being based on the value recorded and the diurnal variation. In truth, all but the most obsessive patients find this irksome and most soon abandon regular recording. There is no doubt that all patients whose asthma is difficult to control should record their PEF twice daily but the need for this in well-controlled patients is less certain.

Action plans

A further extension of the diary and PEF recording is to provide the patient with a written 'Action plan'. There are a wide variety of these, stretching from the simple and practical to those requiring a college degree and a computer for their use! As with all asthma management — the simpler the better. If the action plan occupies more than one typed sheet it will probably not be understood by most patients and its recommendations will not be obeyed. Provided the patient knows the names and correct doses of medications, a simple credit-card-sized Action Plan is very convenient (Fig. 16).

ASTHMA ACTION PLAN

Name: _____
Hospital No: ____ Tel: _____
GP: _____ Tel: _____

MEASURE PEAK FLOW BEFORE RELIEVER

| BEST PEAK FLOW | *500* |

PEAK FLOW	TREATMENT
Below *350*	double dose of preventer
Below *300*	start prednisolone contact doctor
Below *200*	continue reliever dial for ambulance

SYMPTOMS	TREATMENT
Waking from sleep with asthma or needing reliever more than 4 times a day	double dose of preventer
Waking twice or more with asthma or needing reliever more than 6 times daily	start prednisolone contact doctor
Taking prednisolone and needing reliever more than 2 hourly	continue reliever dial for ambulance

Figure 16
Credit card 'Action Plan' indicating how a patient should increase medication with a fall in peak flow or (on the reverse side) a change in symptoms.

The action plan should contain the following elements:

- Expected condition when well controlled, based on symptoms and/or PEF recording
- Indications for simple extra medication, based on symptoms and/or PEF recording
- Indication for emergency treatment, based on symptoms and/or PEF recording
- How to step down treatment when condition improves

Who should take care of the patient and where?

Asthma is a common disease in children and adults and most are only mildly affected. For these patients, excellent care can be provided by the general practitioner or primary care paediatrician. The difficult questions arise when control is not good and the patient is limited in normal everyday activities or when he appears to be resistant to acceptable doses of usual medication. In such patients it would be worth obtaining the opinion of an expert in adult or paediatric respiratory medicine, who should also have access to a well-equipped lung function laboratory. Once the patient has been stabilized, further supervision will depend upon the circumstances and experience of the various physicians involved. The potential for serious side-effects means that most steroid-dependent children and all patients taking high doses of inhaled or oral steroids should be seen at a specialist clinic.

When should the patient be sent straight to the Accident and Emergency Department?
- If the patient has bad asthma which is getting worse, despite treatment
- If the patient is cyanosed or drowsy
- If the patient is scared
- If the doctor is scared!

Appendix
Doses of asthma medications and
PEF measurements

Regular maintenance medication
Bronchodilators

Salbutamol
Short-acting inhaled β_2-agonist for symptom relief
Syrup for small children — 0.15 mg/kg/dose (max 3 mg) up to 4 times daily
Nebulizer solution (5 mg/ml) — 0.5 ml diluted to 2–3 ml up to 4 times daily
MDI (100 µg/puff) with or without spacer — 1–2 puffs as needed up to 4
  times daily
Dry powder inhaler (Diskhaler/Diskus) — 200 or 400 µg, 1–2 as needed
  up to 4 times daily

Terbutaline
Short-acting inhaled β_2-agonist for symptom relief
Syrup for small children — 0.15 mg/kg/dose (max 3 mg) up to 4 times daily
Nebulizer solution (10 mg/ml) — 0.5 ml diluted to 2–3 ml up to 4 times daily
MDI (250 µg/puff) with or without spacer — 1–2 puffs as needed up to 4
  times daily
Dry powder inhaler (Turbohaler) — (500 µg/dose; 200 µg/dose available
  on some markets) — 1 inhalation up to 4 times daily

Fenoterol
Short-acting inhaled β_2-agonist for symptom relief
MDI (100 µg/puff) — 1–2 puffs as needed up to 4 times daily
MDI (200 µg/puff) — only indicated occasionally

Salmeterol
Long-acting β_2-agonist for regular use
MDI (25 µg/puff) — 1–2 puffs twice daily
Dry powder inhaler (Diskhaler/Diskus) — (50 µg/puff) — 1–2 puffs twice
  daily

Formoterol (eformoterol fumarate)
Long-acting inhaled β_2-agonist for regular use
Dry powder inhaler (12 µg/capsule) — 1–2 capsules twice daily
Dry powder inhaler (Turbohaler) — 6–12 µg twice daily

Bambuterol
Long-acting oral β_2-agonist for regular use
10–20 mg at bedtime

Cont'd.

Other β₂-agonists

Pirbuterol, reproterol, orciprenaline, rimiterol

These are used less often

> **Note**: It is not recommended to prescribe regular daily short-acting β-agonist medication on a long-term basis and these drugs should be used primarily as *rescue medication*. Salmeterol and formoterol should only be used in combination with inhaled steroids

Ipratropium bromide

Anticholinergic bronchodilator, less effective than β-agonists in routine asthma treatment

Nebulizer solution (0.25 mg/ml) — 0.25–1.00 ml 3–4 times daily

MDI (20/40 µg/puff) — 1–2 puffs 3–4 times daily

Dry powder inhaler (20-40 µg/capsule) — 1–2 capsules 3–4 times daily

Oxitropium bromide

MDI (100 µg/puff) — 2 puffs 3 times daily

Combination bronchodilator inhalers

Combivent:

MDI: ipratropium bromide (20 µg) and salbutamol (100 µg) — 2 puffs 4 times daily

Nebulizer: ipratropium bromide (500 µg) and salbutamol (2.5 mg) in 2.5 ml 3 to 4 times daily

Duovent

MDI: ipratropium bromide (220 µg) and fenoterol (100 mg) — 1–2 puffs 3 to 4 times daily

Nebulizer: ipratropium bromide (500 µg) and salbutamol (1.25 mg) in 4 ml 3 to 4 times daily

Inhaled steroids

Low-dose (BDP beclomethasone): total daily dose < 800 µg in adults, 400 µg in children

High-dose (BDP beclomethasone): 800–2000 µg in adults, 400–1000 µg in children

- Dose delivered to lungs depends on delivery device
- Daily dose determined by asthma severity; use lowest dose needed to maintain control
- Twice daily administration recommended

Beclomethasone dipropionate

MDI (50, 100, 200 and 250 µg/puff)
Dry powder inhaler (100, 200 and 400 µg/dose)

Budesonide

MDI (50 and 200 µg/puff)
Dry powder inhaler (Turbohaler) — (100, 200 and 400 µg/inhalation)
Nebulized (250 µg/ml; 500 µg/ml;1–2 mg twice daily)

Fluticasone propionate

MDI (25, 50, 125 and 250 µg/puff)
Dry powder inhaler (Diskus) — (50, 100, 250 and 500 µg/dose)
Approximately twice as potent as beclomethasone and budesonide

Parenteral steroids

Use lowest dose possible for adequate control
Adults: give as single morning dose
Children: use alternate morning single dose (average maintenance dose
  up to 1 mg/kg/alternate day for prednisolone)
Prednisolone (1 and 5 mg; enteric-coated tablets also available)
Deflazacort (6 mg tablets)
Triamcinolone acetonide (40 mg/ml) — intramuscular injection 1–2 ml

Other controllers

Sodium cromoglycate

Nebulizer solution — 20 mg (2 ml) 3–4 times daily as prophylaxis
Powder inhaler (Spinhaler) — 20 mg 3–4 times daily as prophylaxis
MDI (5 mg/puff) — 1–2 puffs 4 times daily as prophylaxis

Nedocromil sodium

MDI (2 mg/puff) — 2 puffs 2–4 times daily as prophylaxis

Montelukast (an antileukotriene)

Tablet (10 mg adult, 5 mg children aged 6–14 years — once daily in
  evening) as prophylaxis

Slow-release theophylline preparations

Many preparations as prophylaxis
Children: build up to about 5 mg/kg twice daily with checks on blood level
Adults: build up to about 4 mg/kg twice daily with checks on blood level
  (*NB*: These doses are designed to give blood levels in the range of
  5–10 mg/l)

Short ('crash') course of corticosteroids

Children: Oral prednisolone — start with 2.0 mg/kg/day in divided doses and reduce in steps to zero over 5–10 days provided control is adequate. If not, consider higher dose or longer course but courses lasting more than 2–3 weeks are likely to cause side-effects

Adults: Similar to children, but start with prednisolone about 30–40 mg/day and reduce over 7–10 days. Oral steroids may be stopped abruptly rather than tailed down if preferred

Acute (emergency) medications

Bronchodilators

Salbutamol
Nebulized:
Children — 0.15 mg/kg up to 5.0 mg maximum diluted to 2–3 ml with normal saline
Adults — 5.0 mg diluted to 2–3 ml with normal saline
Both — 20 puffs of MDI into large volume spacer
Intravenous:
Children — 0.1–0.2 µg/kg/min
Adults — initially 5 µg/min, then adjust to avoid excessive heart rate response (average 3–20 µg/min)

Terbutaline
Nebulized:
Children — 0.3 mg/kg up to 10 mg maximum, diluted to 2–3 ml with normal saline
Adults — 10 mg diluted to 2–3 ml with normal saline
Both — 20 puffs of MDI into large volume spacer
Intravenous:
Children — 0.02–0.06 µg/kg/min
Adults — 1.5–5.0 µg/min

Ipratropium bromide
Nebulized:
To be added to β_2-agonist inhalation every 2–4 hours
Children — 5–7 µg/kg
Adults — 500 µg (2 ml of 250 µg/ml solution)

Aminophylline

If patient has not been taking theophylline preparations; loading dose of 7 mg/kg up to maximum of 250 mg over 20 min then maintenance of 0.5–1.0 mg/kg/hr and measure blood level

If patient has been taking theophylline preparations: no loading dose, only maintenance of 0.5–1.0 mg/kg/hr and measure blood level

Corticosteroids

Oral prednisolone

Children: give 2 mg/kg stat, then tail down over 7–10 days
Adults: 60 mg stat, then tail down over 7–10 days

Intravenous hydrocortisone

Children: 4 mg/kg every 6 hours
Adults: 200 mg every 6 hours

Intravenous methylprednisolone .

Children: 1–1.5 mg/kg every 6 hours
Adults: 100 mg every 6 hours

PEF in normal children related to height

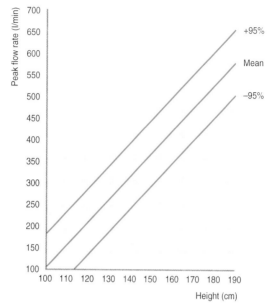

Figure 17

*This nomogram results from tests carried out by Professor S Godfrey and his colleagues on a sample of 382 normal boys and girls aged 5 to 18 years. Each child blew 5 times into a standard Wright Peak Flow Meter and the highest reading was accepted in each case. All measurements were completed within a 6-week period. The outer lines of the graph indicated that the results of 95% of the children fell within these boundaries. (Redrawn from Godfrey et al, Br J Dis Chest (1970) **64**: 15.)*

Normal peak flow readings in adults

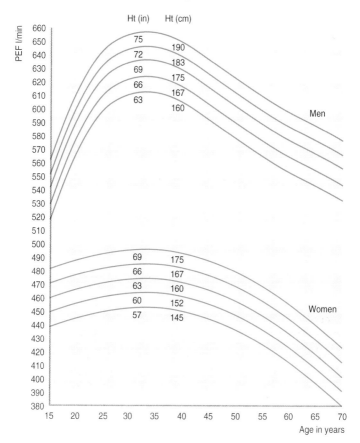

Figure 18
Peak expiratory flow in normal subjects. Standard deviation men = 48 litres/min, standard deviation women = 42 litres/min. In men values of PEF up to 1000 litres/min less than predicted, and in women less than 85 litres/min less than predicted, are within normal limits. (Redrawn from Gregg I, Nunn AJ, Br Med J (1973) 3: 282)

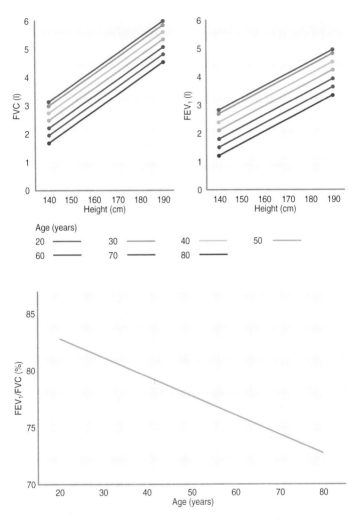

Figure 19
Normal values for FVC and FEV_1 in adult men and their ratio to each other. From the Working Party on Standardisation of Lung Function Tests of the European Community for Steel and Coal. Eur Respir J **6**: Suppl 16, 1993.

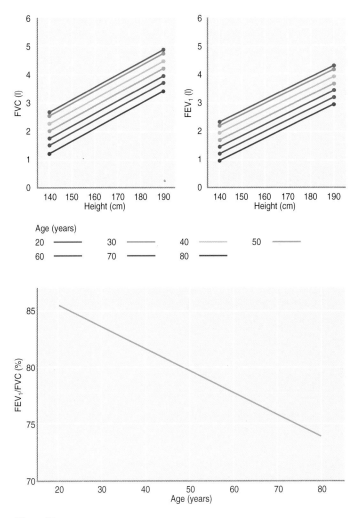

Figure 20
Normal values for FVC and FEV$_1$ in adult women and their ratio to each other.
From the Working Party on Standardisation of Lung Function Tests of the
European Community for Steel and Coal. Eur Respir J **6**: Suppl 16, 1993.

Index

Suggested reading

Asthma: a follow-up statement from an international paediatric asthma consensus group (1992) *Arch Dis Child* **67**: 240–8.

Barnes PJ. (1996) Pathophysiology of asthma. *Br J Clin Pharmacol* **42**: 3–10.

Barnes PJ (1996) New drugs for asthma. *Clin Exp Allergy* **26**: 738–45.

Barnes PJ, Grunstein MM, Leff A, Woolcock AJ, eds (1997) *Asthma,* Philadelphia: Lippencott-Raven.

Barnes PJ, Pedersen S, Busse W (1998) Efficacy and safety of inhaled steroids in asthma. *Am J Respir Crit Care Med* **157** (suppl).

Barnes PJ, Chung KF, Evans TW et al, eds (1994) *Therapeutics in Respiratory Disease*, p. 174. Edinburgh: Churchill Livingstone.

Barnes PJ, Rodger IW, Thomson NC, eds (1998) *Asthma: Basic Mechanisms and Clinical Management*, 3rd edn, London: Academic Press.

British Thoracic Society (1997) Guidelines on the management of asthma. *Thorax* **52** (suppl): S1–2.

Clark TJH, Godfrey S, Lee TH (1999) *Asthma,* 4th edn.

Global Initiative on Asthma.

Godfrey S, Bar–Yishay E (1993) Exercise-induced asthma revisited. *Respir Med* **87**: 331–44.